Essential Oils

The complete guide to using essential oils for aromatherapy, weight loss, and more!

Table Of Contents

Introduction 1

Chapter 1: Essential Oil Basics 2

Chapter 2: Aromatherapy and Fragrance 7

Chapter 3: Weight Loss 11

Chapter 4: Skin and Hair Care 13

Chapter 5: Household Use....................................20

Conclusion 22

Introduction

I want to thank you and congratulate you for downloading the book, *"Essential Oils"*.

This book contains helpful information about essential oils, and how you can use them for a range of benefits!

Essential oils can be used in a variety of ways, for a large range of different benefits.

Aromatherapy is a common method of use, and this will be discussed in length in this book.

You will soon discover how to use different essential oils to improve and alleviate medical conditions, ease stress, improve health, and even to clean the house!

Essential oils are a great natural alternative to many medical treatments, and to commercial cleaners.

This book will explain to you tips and techniques that will allow you to successfully use essential oils for this large range of benefits, all from the comfort of your home.

Thanks again for downloading this book, I hope you enjoy it!

Chapter 1:
Essential Oil Basics

Essential oils are the distilled essences of plants. They are hydrophobic substances, i.e. water repelling, which is why they are commonly called oils; however they are not the same as true oils like olive or coconut oil. Chemists consider true oils to contain fatty acids. Essential oils do not contain these fats. Further, though they are hydrophobic, they do not necessarily feel oily. Some essential oils are light and have the viscosity and appearance of water.

To explain the concept of a distilled plant essence, imagine a plant or a part of it like the leaves, stems or roots. Plants are roughly comprised of fibrous material, water, and their nutrients. The nutrients, which we can call its essence, provide us with whatever advantage this plant is proven to provide. For example, lavender flowers are proven to have antibacterial properties. If we take away the fibrous material and water, what we would be left with are the antibacterial substances.

It is this essence which makes a particular plant different from other plants. All plants basically share the same chemical make-up: fibrous material for its structure and water for its moisture. Only their essences differ. This is why the term 'essential oil' is very accurate. It is considered 'oil' because it is hydrophobic, and it is called 'essential' because it is the essence of the plant.

Since plants are comprised mostly of fibrous material and water, you need a lot of them to create even just an ounce of essential oil. For example, you need 100 pounds of lavender flowers to make 1 pound of lavender oil. The amount of plants or plant parts you need depends on how much essence there naturally is in them. Roses have less essential oil per flower compared to lavender which is why 4000 pounds are needed to create 1 pound. This is why essential oils are expensive. In addition, the process of distillation is difficult and time-consuming.

However, since essential oils are very concentrated, you only need to use a small amount every time you use them. Although they are one of the most expensive liquids per ounce, they become inexpensive when it comes to how they are used.

It is a mistake to think that the use of essential oils is a hippie invention which eschews the science of modern medicine. It is also a mistake to think that essential oils only have a placebo effect. Actually, modern medicine acknowledges the effectivity of essential oils for minor illnesses. Though the knowledge of essential oils was not arrived at scientifically, years of experience have proven that they are indeed effective. In the past, natural healers have discovered through trial and error that certain plants have healing properties. Since they still did not have the technology of distillation, they used the crushed whole plant or brewed teas from them. In time, when distillation was discovered, people were able to create essential oils.

When buying and using essential oils, here are some pointers to keep in mind:

- Make sure that you are buying true essential oil and not artificial fragrance oil. The latter is merely oil that is artificially scented. While they can replace essential oils for scenting a room, the scent will be inferior. Those who are used to the scent of true essential oils will notice a difference in scent quality. Also, never use artificial fragrance oils for your skin or hair. Besides not gaining any advantage from it, these might cause irritation for sensitive folks. Remember that the advantage of essential oils comes from the fact that they are distilled plant essences. You are after the plant essence and not simply the scent. Further, never *ever* ingest artificial fragrance oils.

- To be sure that you are buying true essential oils, buy from reputable sources which properly label all of their products. They should be able to tell you the manufacture date and country of origin for each essential oil.

- You don't have to buy organic essential oils unless you are particularly sensitive to inorganic produce. Organic essential oils can be double or triple the price of inorganic brands.

- Be wary of brands which sell different essential oils for the same price. They are likely fake. Remember that the quantity of plants needed to make each kind of essential oil differs depending on how much essence each plant naturally contains. For example, rose essential oil must be more expensive than lavender oil.

- Buy only the amount of essential oil you can use within 5 years or so. Dark, viscous oils made from wood or stems can last for 5-10 years. Those made from flowers can last about 3-5 years while those made from citrus fruits will only last a year or less. Sniff the essential oil and take note of that fragrance. Once the scent changes, the product has expired. Do not attempt to use it or you might experience adverse effects. You should treat expired essential oils as you would expired medicines and cosmetics.

- Essential oils are stored in opaque glass bottles to keep the light out, but all the same, keep them in a dark, cool place to preserve their quality.

- Some essential oils can be used for various purposes. For example, lavender can be used for fragrance, aromatherapy, topical skin care, and even for cooking and household cleaning. If you need something for all these purposes, it can be cheaper to buy this in a bulk container, rather than in smaller bottles.

- While some essential oils are multi-purpose, there will be oils which are more effective than others. For example, both lavender and tea tree oils are good for acne, but tea tree oil is more effective, i.e. it will provide faster results or it is the better choice for severe cases. What you choose to get in the end will depend on your personal preferences and budget.

- Generally speaking, lavender essential oil is the best multi-purpose oil for beginners. It is also the safest to use. It can be used for children, pregnant and nursing women, and even for pets.

- Regarding safety, do not assume that as long as something is natural it is safe, non-irritating or non-poisonous. Remember that many of the irritants and poisons known to man are natural like poison ivy, oak, jelly fish, and snake venom. While some essential oils can be ingested, some must be limited to topical use. Some essential oils are effective for household purposes but can be poisonous when inhaled. In this book, we will discuss only those essential oils which are generally safe for topical use and inhalation.

- Even if an essential oil is generally safe, it can still cause irritation if you have sensitive skin or have allergies. You should always do a skin test when using essential oils topically, and you should start with the smallest quantity when using it as a fragrance or for aromatherapy. We will discuss how to do this in the succeeding chapters.

- If you are pregnant, nursing, or suffer from any medical conditions like asthma or high blood pressure, avoid essential oils, or only use a small amount. Be very cautious and read the labels and guidelines for each individual oil.

Chapter 2:
Aromatherapy and Fragrance

Aromatherapy is exactly what it sounds like – using aroma as therapy. Certain aromas or scents can improve your mood, reduce stress, increase concentration and relax you. Consider how you react when you smell certain scents. Your reaction to the smell of flowers will be different from your reaction to the smell of garbage. If you are in a foul mood, smelling garbage will more than likely darken your day, while smelling flowers will more than likely improve your mood.

The key word to keep in mind here is 'likely.' If you are in a foul mood and deliberately insist on frowning, no amount of pleasant scent will improve your mood; but if you allow the scent to affect you then you will likely sense your mood gradually improving.

The way aromatherapy works is a psychological process which depends on how the brain instinctively responds to various stimuli. It is similar to the way certain kinds of music can relax or stimulate the mind. Humans instinctively feel better when they smell pleasant fragrances and automatically frown when they smell something foul, but since humans are more than just instinct, we can choose to reject what our bodies are telling us. Thus, we can choose to ignore hunger and other instinctual urgings.

That said, aromatherapy will be much more effective if you allow it to have an effect on you. However, we must always be reasonable with our expectations. A person who is battling severe clinical depression cannot expect aromatherapy alone to completely cure the problem; but for normal people battling occasional stress, aromatherapy can be a big help.

To use essential oils for aromatherapy, you need to choose your preferred method for distributing the scent. Here are some of your choices and their advantages and disadvantages.

Methods:

1. **Electric diffuser** – follow the instructions provided with each machine. Always dilute the essential oil with an equal amount of water. Directly burning the oil will alter its scent. Never leave the machine alone for long periods of time, or else use a machine with a built in timer.

2. **Oil burner** – use a tea light to heat the diluted oil. Never burn the oil for longer than 2 hours at a time. Blow out the candle when the water has evaporated. Never add more water to hot essential oil.

3. **Scented candle** – use like any candle. Avoid cheap candles which might not contain enough essential oil to create a scent.

4. **Scented potpourri** – start with 10 drops of essential oil for each cup of potpourri. Use more or less depending on how intense you would like the scent to be.

5. **Room spray** – you can either buy this or make your own. To make your own, mix 10 drops of essential oil with ½ cup distilled water and ½ cup 100 proof vodka. Keep this solution in a glass or plastic spray bottle. Shake well before using.

6. **Direct sniffing or scented handkerchief** – sniff the scent directly from the bottle or place a few drops on your handkerchief.

7. **Scented massage oil or body fragrance** – add 10 drops to 1 cup of massage oil. See recipes below for body fragrance. Do not do this if you have a sensitive nose. Also, make sure that your skin is not sensitive to the essential oil when using it for massage or as a fragrance.

Body fragrance recipes:

- **Pure essential oil as a fragrance** – apply 1 drop of pure essential oil (or a combination of oils) to pulse points. Do not do this is you have sensitive skin. This provides the most intense scent.

- **Solid fragrance** – mix ¼ cup of melted beeswax with 15-25 drops of essential oil. Pour boiling water into a glass jar or metal tin to sterilize it, pour the water out then allow the jar or tin to dry. Pour the liquid beeswax into the container and allow to cool before using. This is good for travellers since it does not spill.

- **Oil fragrance** – mix 4 ounces of neutral smelling oil like jojoba or grape seed with 10-15 drops of essential oil. Jojoba or grape seed oil easily absorbs into the skin. This is a good choice for those who dislike the waxy residue of solid fragrances. The scent intensity is the same as for solid fragrances.

- **Body spray** – follow the recipe for room spray described above. This provides the most subtle scent. If you are sensitive to alcohol, use more water but make sure that you shake the product for a longer time. Since essential oils are hydrophobic, the alcohol allows it to be evenly distributed in the water base, but shaking it very well will have the same effect.

Once you have chosen your method, choose your preferred scent according to your needs:

Relaxing/stress reducing – lavender, jasmine, vanilla, chamomile, rose, sandalwood, ylang-ylang

Possible combinations for variety:

1. 1:1:1 ratio of lavender, jasmine and vanilla

2. 1:1 ratio of chamomile and rose

3. 1:3 ratio of sandalwood and rose

Stimulating/for increasing concentration – peppermint, cinnamon, eucalyptus, ginger, basil, clove, citrus scents like lemon, lime and grapefruit

Possible combinations for variety:

1. 1:1 ratio of ginger and lemon

2. 1:1 ratio of peppermint and basil

3. 1:2 ratio of clove and cinnamon

Chapter 3:
Weight Loss

Before we begin to discuss the use of essential oils for weight loss, we must make an important clarification: essential oils can help with your weight loss efforts but they cannot replace a reduced-calorie diet and regular exercise. Essential oils help by reducing the appetite, and slightly increasing the metabolism.

Here are the essential oils you can use for weight loss: lemon, grapefruit, cinnamon, ginger, peppermint.

You can use essential oils for weight loss through the aromatherapy methods described above, or through ingestion. The former will help to decrease your appetite while the latter will slightly increase your metabolism.

When you choose to ingest essential oils, you have to be *absolutely sure* that you are using true essential oil and not artificial fragrance oil. If you are in doubt, then don't ingest it. For this purpose, it is better to buy essential oils from cooking supply stores just to be on the safe side.

When ingesting essential oils, limit yourself to 2 drops a day. If you have never done this before, start with 1 drop for the first week just to see if you will experience any discomfort or allergies. If you do, then you should stop and just limit yourself to aromatherapy methods. If you don't experience any adverse effects, then increase your consumption to 2 drops.

Here are some ways to ingest essential oils:

- Add 1-2 drops to a glass of water. It is better to do this in the morning right after you wake up.

- Add to a cup of hot tea. Lemon, peppermint and ginger are good choices for this.

- Use to flavor baked goods. Lemon, cinnamon and ginger are especially good for sweet items like muffins.

- Use cinnamon to flavor oatmeal or other cereals, hot milk or hot chocolate.

- Add lemon or grapefruit to salad dressings. Make sure that you add only 1-2 drops per serving.

Chapter 4:
Skin and Hair Care

When using essential oils for skin or hair ailments, you can apply it pure, or diluted with carrier oil. Carrier oil is any kind of true oil, i.e. one that contains fatty acids like olive or coconut oil, which is supposed to dilute or 'carry' the essential oil. Recall that essential oils are hydrophobic so they cannot be diluted with water.

Using undiluted essential oils will provide the most benefits, but they can be irritating. To check if you can use pure oil or must dilute it, do a skin test. First, apply 1 drop of pure oil to a hidden part of the skin, like the inner elbow or behind the ear. Wait 24 hours to see if irritation occurs. If it does, wash it off immediately with water. Repeat the test with 1 drop of oil diluted with an equal amount of carrier oil. If irritation still occurs, repeat the test with 1 drop of oil and 2 drops of carrier oil. If irritation still occurs, find another solution. It is possible that you are sensitive or allergic to one essential oil but not to another. For sensitive individuals, it is best to start with lavender oil which is the gentlest and safest for even the most sensitive individuals. If lavender does not work for you, it may be best to completely avoid using essential oils.

If you can use pure essential oil, apply it directly to the affected areas. Never use pure essential oils near the sensitive eye area.

If you need to dilute essential oils, either combine them beforehand and store the solution in an opaque bottle or combine them together in a small bowl or on your palm every time you need it. If you keep your solution in a bottle, shake it to ensure that it is perfectly mixed. Make sure that you use the correct ratio based on the results of your skin test, e.g. 1:1 or

1:2 essential oil to carrier oil. Use the essential oil as you would a moisturizer or ointment.

Your choice of carrier oil will depend on your skin type. Here are some good choices:

Dry or mature skin – olive, avocado, rosehip, argan (choose according to scent)

Normal skin – coconut, jojoba, sweet almond, apricot kernel (choose according to scent, only jojoba smells neutral)

Oily skin – grape seed (oily skin can only use this kind of carrier oil)

If you prefer a cream based product, you can make a cream base, and then mix in your essential oil. Here is a recipe for basic cream base:

- ¼ cup carrier oil

- ¼ cup beeswax (oily skin) or cocoa butter (normal skin) or shea butter (dry or mature skin)

- 10 drops of essential oil

Procedure: Melt the beeswax, cocoa or shea butter over low heat. Remove from the heat then add in the carrier oil. Mix well. When slightly cool, mix in the essential oil. Pour everything in a sterilized glass container then allow to cool completely before use.

Some people like to use a facial toner before applying moisturizer. Here is a recipe for basic toner:

- ¼ cup distilled water or strongly brewed green or black tea (use 1 tea bag with ¼ cup of boiling water.

- 5 drops of essential oil

- *For oily skin only:* 2 tablespoons 100 proof vodka or 2 tablespoons apple cider or white vinegar

Procedure: Pour everything in a sterilized bottle then shake well. Use a cotton ball to apply. Shake well before every use.

Acne

The best essential oils for acne are tea tree, lavender, eucalyptus, and neem oil. They all fight acne-causing bacteria, but your choice will depend on various factors. Tea tree is the most effective against bacteria and is the best choice for severe acne. The rest are less effective but can provide other benefits.

Lavender is the most versatile essential oil. It can be used to reduce stress, to reduce fine lines and wrinkles, and as a body fragrance.

Eucalyptus can be used to stimulate the mind and clear the sinuses when you have a cold.

Neem smells bad, but is best for mature skin when combined with a very emollient oil like olive or avocado oil. This is the best choice for older people who still occasionally break out.

For very big pimples, you can see a major improvement in its size overnight if you dab pure essential oil on it. Do not do this regularly if you are sensitive to pure essential oil.

Acne can also improve with weekly steam facials. To do this, boil 5 cups of water then add 10 drops of essential oil. You can use any of the above except neem which has an unpleasant scent. For variety, you can also use rosemary or lemon oil which can help to reduce oil production. Bend your face over the water, then cover your head to prevent the steam from dissipating.

Acne scars or age spots

Lemon essential oil can help to fade the dark spots left by healed pimples. You can use this together with your acne treatments. Combine equal amounts of lemon oil with any of the suggested oils for acne. It can also help oily skin produce less oil.

For mature skin that tends to be on the dry side, apply pure or diluted lemon oil only on the age spots. Do not apply it all over your face since it can dry the skin. For this specific purpose, rosehip oil is the best carrier oil since it can also help to fade age spots.

Fungal infections

The same essential oils which work for acne can be used to kill fungi. Use coconut oil for this problem since it contains natural anti-fungal properties, or else use pure essential oil if your skin can take it.

Apply the pure or diluted essential oil as you would an ointment. To avoid inadvertently wiping it off, soak a piece of gauze then keep it in place with a bandage.

Insect bites or other itchy patches

Use pure or diluted peppermint or eucalyptus to temporarily relieve itch.

Anti-aging

For relatively young skin, the use of antioxidants can delay the signs of aging. Essential oils of antioxidant rich plants can be used for this purpose. Choose from green tea, jasmine, lemon, grapefruit or orange essential oils.

Possible combinations for variety:

1. 1:1 ratio of green tea and jasmine/lemon

2. 2:1:1 ratio of lemon, grapefruit and orange

Fine lines and wrinkles

Essential oils work against the signs of aging by increasing the blood flow to the face, thus bringing in more nutrients which help to repair and nourish the skin. Lavender, patchouli, rose, sandalwood, and chamomile are good choices for this problem. Choose according to your preferred scent or else make your own combinations.

Possible combinations for variety:

1. 1:1 ratio of lavender and patchouli

2. 1:1 ratio of rose and sandalwood (this provides an intense, feminine scent)

3. 2:1:1 ratio of chamomile, rose and sandalwood (this provides a less intense but still very feminine scent)

4. Use rose essential oil together with rosehip oil for an intensely fragranced product.

Eye area moisturizer

For this purpose, it is better to use carrier oils to dilute your essential oil to avoid irritating the delicate eye area. The carrier oil can be easily patted onto the skin. It will be completely absorbed within a few minutes. Choose the essential oil according to your specific problem, or use equal amounts of each if you suffer from more than 1 problem. Use a 1:2 ratio of essential oil to carrier oil.

Eye wrinkles – rosewood, rose

Puffiness – lemon, rosemary

Dark circles – chamomile

Head lice

Use the same essential oils suggested for acne. Combine 10 drops with ¼ cup of coconut oil, then use this to saturate the whole head. Leave this for at least 15 minutes to kill the lice and loosen nits from the hair shaft, then shampoo off. You might need to repeat this treatment a few times to completely get rid of the problem.

Falling hair

Rosemary and peppermint essential oil are good choices for this problem. You must combine the essential oil with carrier oil to easily apply it to your scalp. Use the carrier oils suggested above according to your hair type, e.g. for dry hair, use the oils suggested for dry skin.

Combine 20 drops of the essential oil with ¼ cup carrier oil. Apply this solution to the scalp with your fingertips. Leave it on for at least an hour or overnight.

You can also combine the essential oil with your shampoo. Use 10 drops per 100 ml. However, this is less effective than the above method.

Chapter 5:
Household Use

If you are the sort who likes to use natural products for cleaning your home, you can use your essential oils. This way, you can avoid the chemicals from commercially available products which may be detrimental to your health in the long run. You can also save money since one bottle of essential oil serves a variety of purposes.

Here are some ideas for how to use essential oils around the home:

Scented dishwashing soap

Add 5-10 drops of your choice of essential oil to 100 ml liquid dishwashing soap. Using one of the suggested relaxing scents can make your dishwashing time a stress relieving experience.

Scented laundry soap

Depending on how fragrant you want your soap to be, use 5-20 drops per 100 grams of laundry soap. Lemon oil is good for brightening whites while tea tree oil is best for disinfecting. Otherwise, choose your essential oil according to your preferred scent.

Disinfecting surfaces

Use lavender or tea tree oil with your cleansing solution. For floors, add 20 drops of essential oil to your bucket of mop water. To make an all-natural disinfectant spray, add 10 drops of essential oil to 100 ml of water or white vinegar and shake well.

Removing mold and mildew

Add 10 drops of tea tree oil to a cup of cleanser, or use the disinfecting spray described above directly on affected areas.

Brightening windows and mirrors

Add 10 drops of lemon oil to 100 ml of water or white vinegar and shake well. Keep this in a spray bottle.

Polishing wood furniture

Melt ¼ cup of beeswax and let it cool for a while. When slightly cool, add 10 drops of lemon oil and mix well. Double this recipe to make your own lemon scented lip balm.

Conclusion

Thank you again for downloading this book!

I hope this book was able to help you learn more about essential oils!

The next step is to put this information to use, and begin using essential oils to improve your health!

Finally, if you enjoyed this book, please take the time to share your thoughts and post a review on Amazon. It'd be greatly appreciated!

Thank you and good luck!

9 781761 030826